MATTHEW DALE

Weight-Lifting Fundamentals

A Simple and Effective Method for Building Strength

First edition

This book was professionally typeset on Reedsy.
Find out more at reedsy.com

I think there are two keys to success. One
is to show up. The other is to keep going.
Most people don't keep going.

-Dan John

Contents

1

Introduction

This book is for anyone looking to get stronger, build muscle, and learn how to program your own workouts with simple and smart programming. This book will also help you gain a solid understanding of the basic principles in strength training. If you have never touched a weight or barbell in your life, this book is for you. If you've been hitting the gym for months, or even years and need some direction to help you become stronger, faster, then this book is for you.

The most important lifts (exercises) we will be learning about are the classic barbell lifts. These are: (the) Squat, Bench Press, Deadlift, Overhead Press, Power Clean, and Snatch. From my own experience in training I can promise you these exercises will give you the most bang for your buck compared to ANY other exercise for gaining strength and becoming stronger.

2

About Me

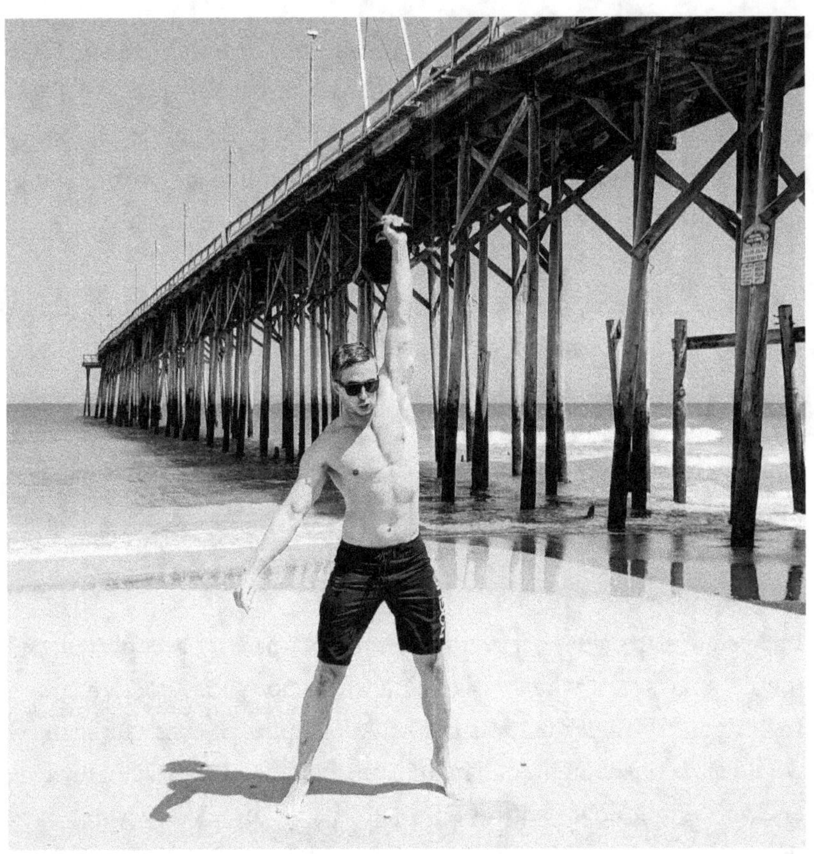

W hy listen to me? What does Matt Dale know about getting stronger? It's my pleasure to tell you about my journey into the strength and health field.

Throughout elementary school and middle school I was a normal looking, average weight and height kid. I was perhaps slightly above average as far as my athleticism and strength goes compared to my other classmates, but not by much. Nothing really stood out. I could skateboard pretty well and that's what I spent most of my time doing from age 10-13.

As a freshman in high-school (2003-2004), online gaming had burst into the scene. This was thanks to high-speed internet becoming available in households. What a joy this was compared to dial up! As the story unfolds, I became addicted to playing Halo 2 online via xbox live with my friends from school and other gamers around the world.

After this phase was over, in 10th grade, I became aware of a new online game that had just come out. It was World of Warcraft. I was mesmerized and became completely sucked into the game as it was another real world I was living in. I'm guessing the age I was (15), the new arrival of high speed internet and online gaming, and the magic of playing with players online was the perfect recipe for a sedentary lifestyle.

I played 8 hours a day on average. And this was after school! I played totally unaware of what I was doing to my body for 2 straight years. In 10th and 11th grade I was hooked on gaming. Never exercising. I would sit at the computer all night, stuffing domino's pizza in my face and washing it down with soda. I bet I barely drank any water back then.

Later in my Junior year a friend made a comment that I was out of breath just by walking to our cars in the student parking lot! And someone in the halls made a comment on my "man boobs". That really sucked. In just 2 short years I went from about 120 lbs and 5'5" as a high-school freshman, to 216 lbs and 6'0" late in my junior year. Granted, I was a growing kid and was bound to gain weight, but this was much more than that.

Once I became hooked on gaming, I had little interest in dating girls. I used to though. From 5 years old to 14 years old, I was always chasing the girls around. But now, going into my senior year of high-school, my interest in women was coming back. The problem was I was so ashamed and embarrassed about my overweight body, that I was afraid to talk to girls anymore. I knew it was time for a change…

The summer going into my senior year I made a decision to start getting healthy. I didn't know hardly anything about fitness, much less weight lifting, but I had to start somewhere. The first thing I remember doing is convincing my mom to buy me a basketball goal for the driveway. It didn't take much convincing as she was more than excited to see me get back outside and off the computer screen. I'd play solo or with my friends. Just looking to get a good sweat. It was the start of something great.

It's funny how you can remember certain things from a long time ago. For some reason, I thought a good weight loss lunch after school was 2 hotdogs without the bun! Senior year I got out at 1:20 and ate lunch at home. I don't know how long i did this for but it's the first dietary change for the good i remember doing while growing up. I know, 2 hotdogs without the bun doesn't sound like the best meal for a healthy lunch… but I've definitely heard of worse!

The next decision I made was to get a bench press. I messed around with it occasionally. I remember benching 200 lbs one time for one rep. It didn't change my life right then and there, but any time spent around weights is a good investment. Years later, it would make a huge impact on me.

Later in my senior year I finally got a girlfriend. I graduated weighing around 190 lbs. I was still a little chunky, but had made much improvement over my 216 lbs junior year self. The summer following graduation I started surfing and skateboarding again. Mainly just being outside and having fun with my friends. And guess what? Just like magic the weight began to melt off. I got all the way down to a lean 158 lbs by the time I was 19!

After realizing I could in fact change my body, I decided to join a gym. I joined the planet fitness that was just a 3 minute drive from my house. I worked out here for 2 or 3 years while I was in college for a computer networking degree. I remember plenty of fun times there with my friends. Sometimes we'd stay for 2 or 3 hours. None of us really knew what we were doing, but we googled some workouts from various online fitness sites and went hard at it!

I was having so much fun working out and lifting weights that upon graduating with my degree, I realized I didn't want to spend my work days stuck behind a computer desk. I had already done that enough in high-school! So I did a big 180 in career choices and decided to be a personal trainer.

I first started out working at a Gold's Gym as a personal trainer. It was okay, but I wanted something different. That's when I decided to build up my home/garage gym piece by piece and train my clients from my own gym. It gave me a lot more freedom in choosing clients and working around my schedule. This was so much more satisfying than keeping only a portion of the payment from working for a corporate gym. To each his own though. Some people like being trainers in big box gyms. I wasn't one of them. The home gym is where I found my calling.

Aside from training clients, my own physical training was starting to take off even more. The year was 2014. At this point, I found some very important mentors to learn from. Two of which are strength coaches and authors named Dan John and Mark Rippetoe. Their work focused on free weights (Barbells, Kettlebells, etc.) They also did a great job at keeping training simple and straight to the point. But keep in mind, simple is not always easy!

It was at this time my own training routine switched from doing every fancy new thing I heard of, to basic full body barbell lifts and kettlebell training. Sure, it might sound boring to do the classic old-school lifts. But guess what? They work like magic. The only barbell exercise I knew how to do before this point was the bench press. All my other exercises were done on machines in the gym and if I was squatting (which was not often) was done on the smith machine.

I began to learn how to squat with the barbell. I had no idea how different it was than squatting inside the smith machine. My balance was definitely tested early on. Learning how to control your body with free weights is obviously good for strength training, but it's also a fantastic way to train your balance. Without balance when squatting weights, you'll fall over.

I'll go into more detail later about the other lifts I started learning about in a couple of chapters. Besides the squat, the other barbell lifts I was introduced to were the deadlift, overhead press, power clean, and snatch. Along with the bench press, these 6 exercises would prove themselves to me that they are truly the KING of strength training. This was the way to get stronger!

3

Before You Start Training

So, you're eager to jump in and start conquering the wights I bet! Well I sure hope so or why else would you be reading this book. Let's start with some basic gym attire and how to dress. If you've already been training for some time, just bare with me for a bit.

I always workout in a t-shirt, gym shorts, and athletic shoes. My favorite overall fitness shoe for the past 10 years has been the Reebok Nano series. They are phenomenal shoes! If it's cold where you are, then sweatpants and a sweatshirt would be a good idea. Just wear those over your shorts/ T shirt and take them off when/if you get too hot.

Next up would be to purchase a high quality lifting belt. The belt not only allows you to lift heavier weights, but also provides much more core stability around your torso and will help protect your back from injury. Think of it as a piece of armor that's wrapping around your midsection. The two belts I recommend are from Bestbelts.net and Roguefitness.com. Best belts is a mom and pops shop located right here in North Carolina. They hand make every belt you order and they're all custom made to your size. If you're looking for a more comfortable belt, I recommend the Rogue USA Nylon Lifting Belt. It's currently $55 from roguefitness.com. It's actually the same belt that 5x Crossfit games champion Mat Fraser uses. If you prefer a more sturdy belt then go with the 3" or 4" wide belt from Best Belts. They're handmade from premium leather and will last you a lifetime. I'm serious. I purchased the 4" Athlete belt from them in 2014 and it's still in my gym bag in 2023. At $110 they're a little more expensive than ones you'd find in a sporting goods store, but it's a wise investment that will help keep you lifting safely for years.

Chalk is a wonderful tool in the weight room. When hands become sweaty, it's difficult to hold on to a heavy barbell weighing several hundred pounds. It keeps your hands dry and allows you to hang on to the bar when you couldn't otherwise. It basically feels like a magic glue of some type.

Another important training accessory for me are my headphones. Lifting weights and listening to your favorite music to get you pumped go hand in hand. Without music, you're kind of alone in your thoughts. The music helps you get that fire going that you might not have had otherwise. And if you don't need music while working out, you're a freak. I'm kidding. Kudos to you. You're a rare breed.

The last things I'll talk about are a gym bag, a light resistance band, and olympic squat shoes. The gym bag is an obvious choice as it will hold all of your training gear, water, phone, etc. The purpose of the resistance band is for warm ups and stretching. The technical term for the ones I like are called "Pull-up assistance bands". It's a single band connected together in a loop. Don't get the ones with handles on them. My favorite and only band I keep in my bag is the "small" type. Every band is the same length, but the sizes vary in width, providing more or less resistance. The small band is roughly ½" in width and provides around 15-35 lbs of resistance. You can get these from Amazon for about $10.

Now for olympic squat shoes. These bad boys have a raised heel on them and are extremely stable. The bottom of the shoe is completely flat and made of hard rubber. The idea is to provide more force into the ground when you are jumping for a power clean or snatch. This is because they aren't squishy like a typical running shoe. They allow much better transfer of power from your feet to the ground. And if you have tight or immobile flexibility in your ankles, you might not be able to properly squat all the way down without your heels coming off the ground. Squat shoes help fix that because of its raised heel. If you've ever seen people squatting in the gym and they place small 5 lb plates under their heels, it's basically serving the function of a squat shoe, but much less efficient. There are several companies with good reputations who make these. I personally have had a pair from Adidas and Nike. Both are great, but I have to take sides and say I like my Nike Romaleo 2's better. These shoes will run you anywhere between $75 and $200. These aren't a must have item right away, but it's worth looking into if you're serious about weight lifting.

4

Home Gym or Public Gym?

Whether you choose to workout at your home gym or at a public gym is completely up to you. Either one will suit your needs in strength training if the proper equipment is in place. Both types of gyms have their pros and cons. Choosing a home gym could come down to various reasons; maybe your schedule is jam packed and you don't have enough time to drive to a gym, or maybe you have some hesitation working out in front of people and would rather workout in private. There are plenty of reasons for selecting either gym.

5

The Home Gym

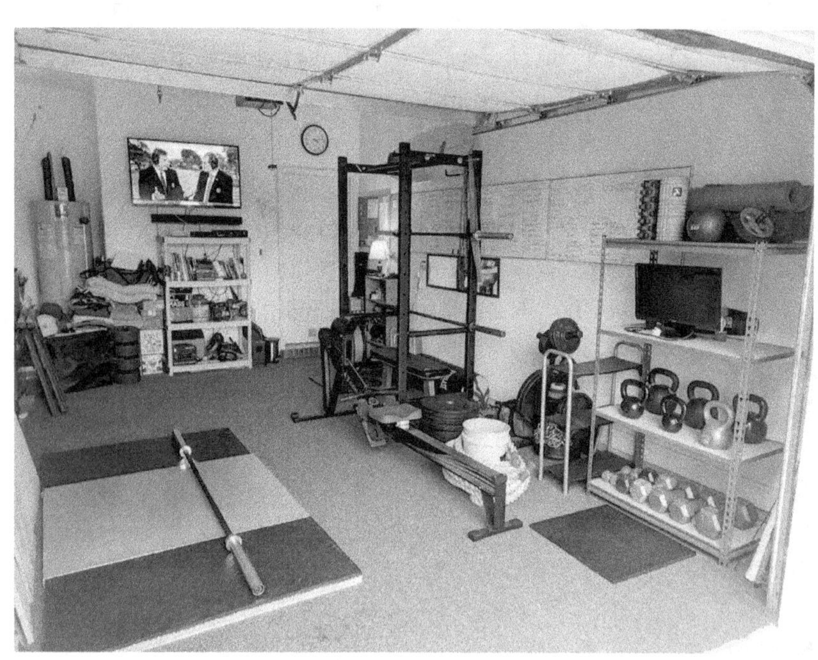

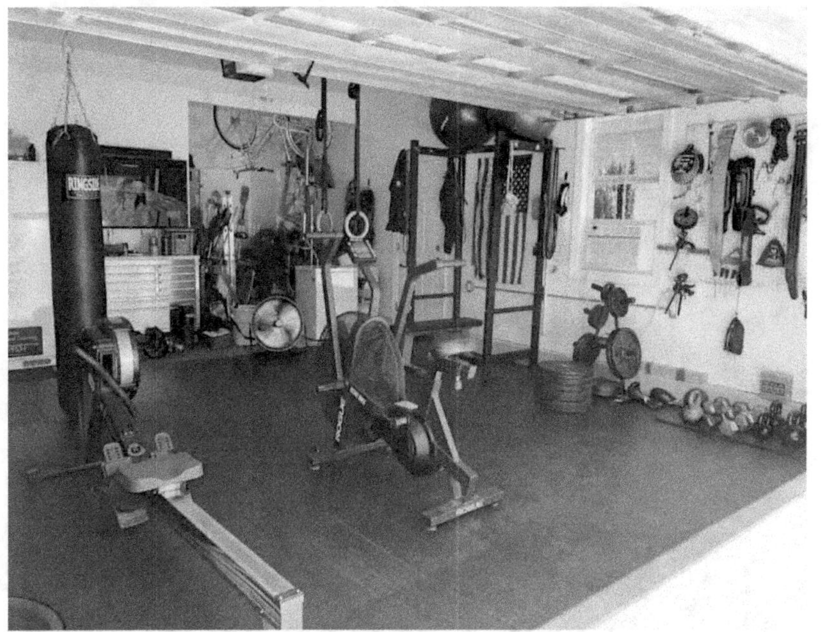

These pictures are 2 of my previous home gyms

Having a nicely equipped home gym is very rewarding. For one, you don't have to drive anywhere to workout. Secondly, you'll never have to wait to use the equipment like you may have to on a busy evening in a public gym. I suppose the main con of a home gym is the initial start up costs for purchasing equipment. But if you shop wisely and use quality equipment, it should last you a long long time. Don't skimp out and go cheap. Trust me, you'll regret it and you'll probably have to re-buy equipment again and again.

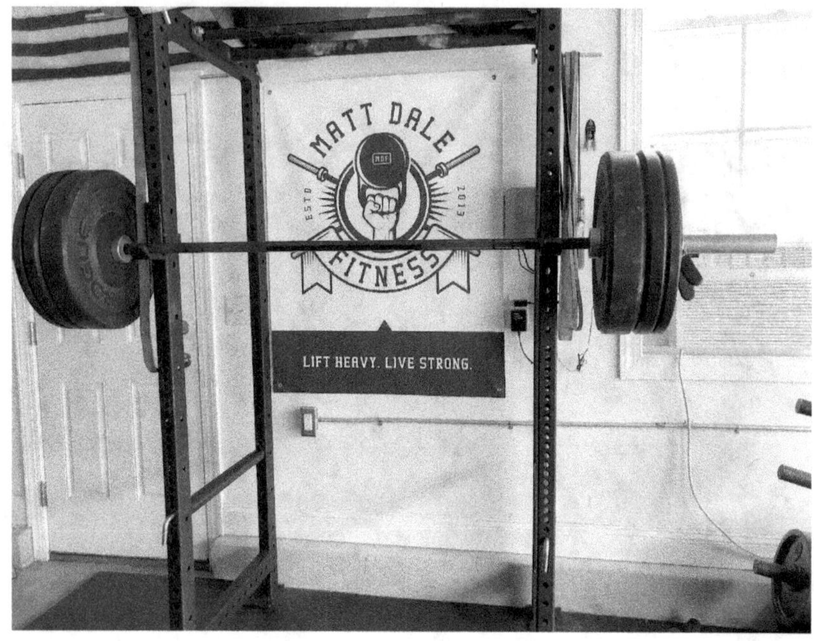

Squat Rack

The first thing you need to buy if you are indeed investing in a home gym is a squat rack. Sometimes called a power rack as well. I've heard people call it a "cage" too. Not only can you perform squats on this, but it will serve as your overhead press and bench press station. I personally have the Rogue R-3 rack (pictured above) and absolutely love it! If you want a slightly cheaper option, a company called Titan Fitness makes some decent equipment for the price. A good rack will also have a built in chin-up bar across the top. You can do so many different things on a rack.

Secondly, you'll need a quality barbell. This is the main piece of equipment you'll be using to get stronger so I recommend getting a good one. Again, Rogue Fitness is hard to beat in terms of quality and price. Next up you'll need some olympic plate weights to progressively load your barbell. You can cheap out on these a little bit and find some decent used ones at a used sporting goods store or buy them secondhand online from craigslist or something similar. If you have the money to spend, I highly recommend getting a set of bumper plates. 2 x 45 lbs, 2 x 25 lbs, and 2 x 10 lbs. These will allow you to perform power cleans and snatches and won't break the floor beneath you when you drop the weights from overhead (which is common practice in the power clean and snatch)

Lastly, you need to get a flat bench to lay down on for bench pressing. You don't have to spend a fortune on these. Either shop on Amazon, Titan Fitness, or Rogue Fitness and you'll find what you need. Another great thing to build into a home gym is a set of wooden gymnastic rings. These are affordable, extremely versatile, and quite easy to install into a garage ceiling. I also recommend getting a weight sled if you have the extra cash. These are great for training your legs and it has a wonderful built in cardio training effect.

If you're looking for a cardio machine to place in your garage gym, I would suggest a rowing machine such as the Concept 2 Rower. It provides a full body warmup. Another machine to consider is the fan bike, such as the Rogue Echo Bike. In addition to pedaling with your legs, these have handle bars that allow you to push and pull, giving you another full body warm up.

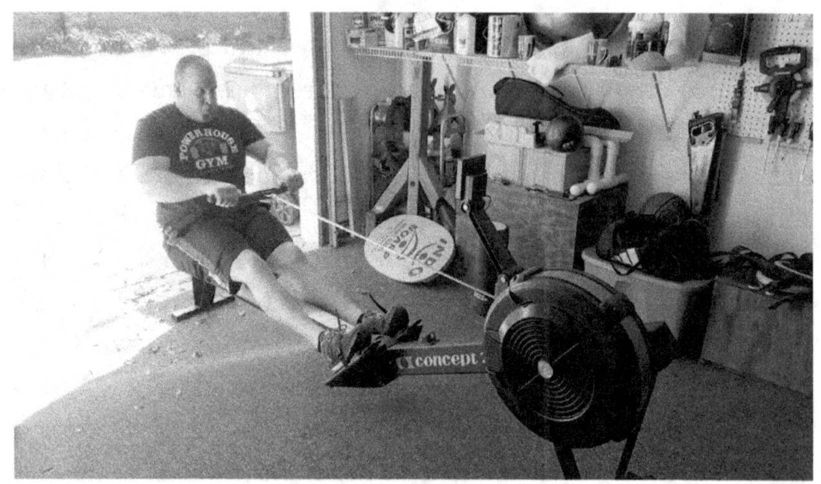

Concept 2 Rower

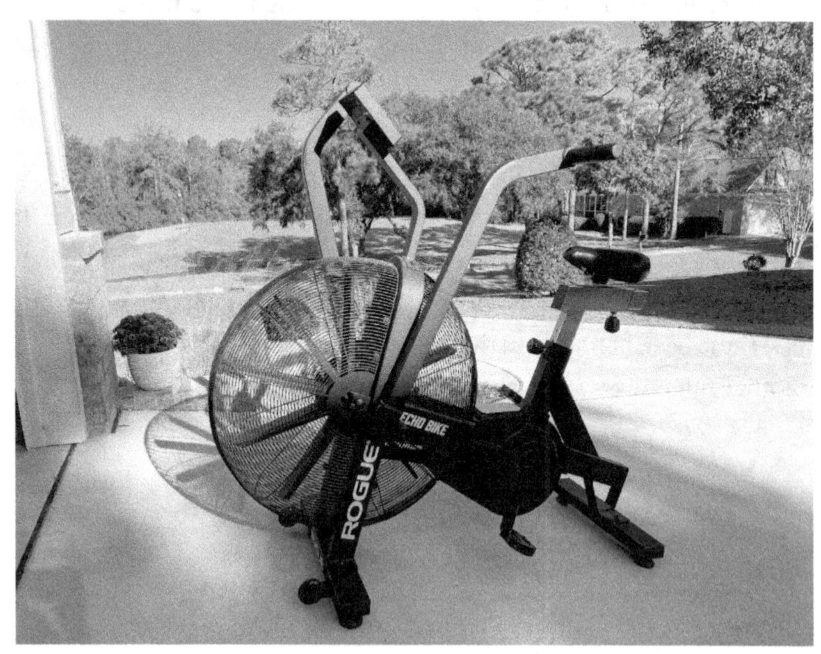

Rogue Echo Bike

6

The Public Gym

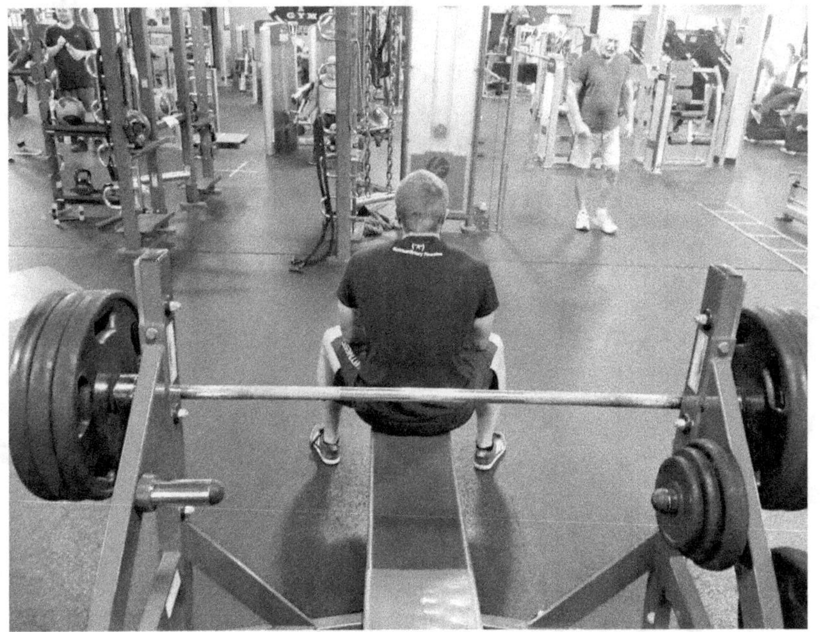

Myself mentally preparing for a heavy bench set

This section doesn't need nearly as much explaining. Choosing a public gym will come down to: it's location, the equipment inside, and the atmosphere of its members. You obviously don't want to join a gym that is 40 miles from your house or you'll always find an excuse not to go. Try to find one that isn't too far from you. Next, take a tour of any gym you're interested in joining. Don't just sign up blindly. Make sure it has the racks, barbells and free weights that you need for strength training. One big no no is choosing planet fitness. They are not free weight friendly and don't have any free weight squat racks or bench presses. It's all machines at planet fitness. Don't get me wrong, it's a decent gym for exercising. But strength training and general exercising are completely different things.

Lastly, when choosing a public gym to join you'll want to take note of the kinds of members working out there. If you feel an off vibe when doing a gym tour and don't like the general attitude of its members or staff, keep looking for a better gym! There are plenty of them these days.

7

Why The Barbell?

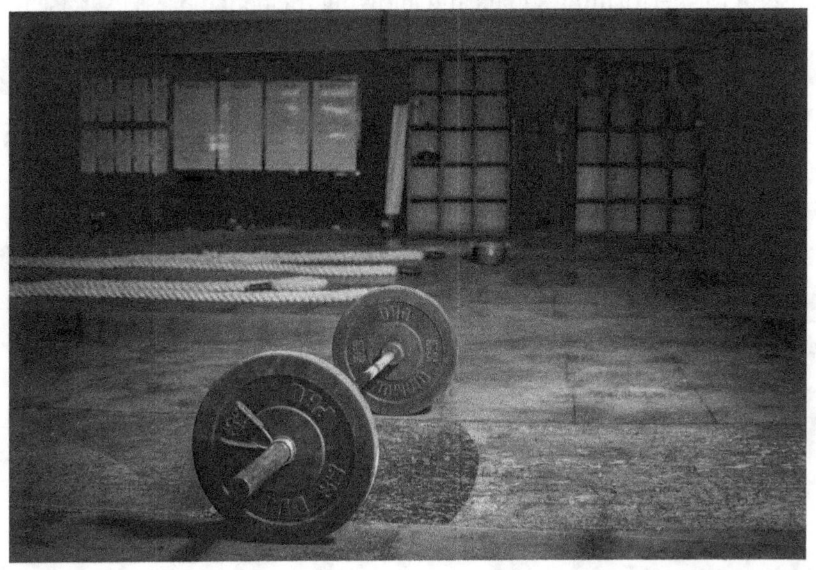

What's so special about the "Barbell"? Well for one, it's one of the oldest pieces of strength equipment ever made. Do you think there were fancy machines and cables and pulleys in a gym 100 years ago? Not hardly. Actually, at this time the now famous bench press exercise didn't even exist. So what did people do? They loaded plates onto a barbell lying on the floor. They picked it up (the Deadlift). They picked it up and jumped the bar to their shoulders (the Power Clean). And they pressed the bar over their heads (the overhead press). Essentially, all that was available to them was picking up weights off the floor and pressing them overhead.

The squat/power rack would come into invention sometime after. Before this point, to barbell squat you'd have to power clean the weight to your shoulders, press it overhead, and carefully lower it behind your head onto your upper back/traps. Talk about a workout! But once people started getting innovative, the rack would prove itself extremely useful for performing squats and allowing the bench press exercise to get started as well.

The barbell is so great because of its versatility and simplicity. And to get stronger, you just simply add small weight increments over time. A standard barbell weighs 45 lbs. They're very sturdy and durable, and a piece of cake to maintain. I can't think of any other piece of gym equipment that allows you to train your entire body as well as the barbell. Now, just because it's simple or seems basic, doesn't mean you need to find newer and fancier trendy exercises. This is a common downfall of so many people in the fitness community. Have faith in the barbell and you will be rewarded greatly!

8

The Big 6 Barbell Lifts

The Squat

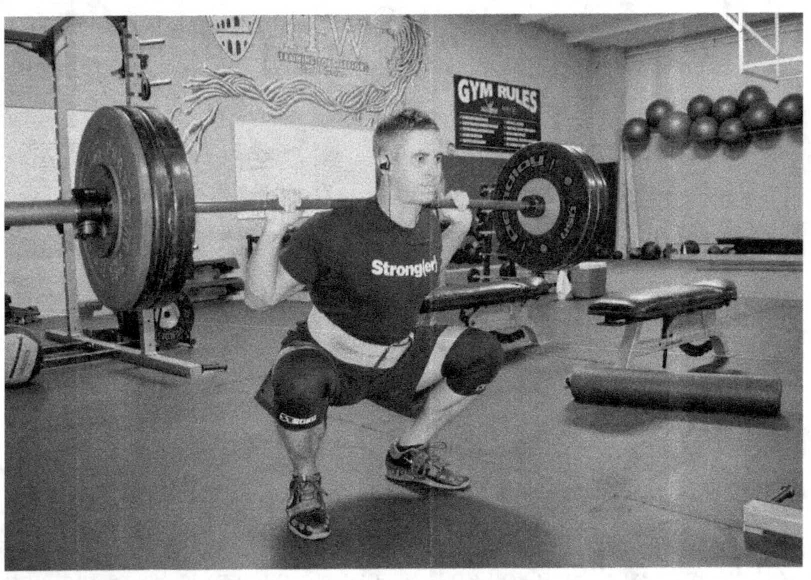

The squat is perhaps the most important exercise there is. No other exercise trains your leg strength as tremendously as the barbell squat does. And not only does it make your legs stronger, it also trains your balance and core muscles. Without a strong core, you'd simply fall and crumble underneath the weights. It's science and makes perfect sense but it seems not many people realize you can train your abs to a large degree just by squatting.

To squat with the barbell, start by setting up an empty bar in a power rack/squat rack. Adjust the J-hooks (the things that hold the barbell to the rack) so you have to squat 3 to 6" underneath the bar in order to get it out of the rack. Don't make the crucial mistake of having your bar too high on the rack. When you're exhausted from squatting a heavy set of 5 reps with 315lbs, the last thing you want is to be unable to re-rack your bar because you set the j-hooks to high. I've seen pretty bad endings when someone is trying with all their might on their tippy toes trying to re-rack the weight and they just can't do it. Lower is always better when choosing how high you should set up your j-hooks for squatting.

Another safety tip is to use the safety spotter arms on the rack. Most racks have adjustable arms you can set to different heights to catch the bar in case you fail to complete a lift.

Okay, so you have your bar set up on the rack, and you're ready to squat. Now, walk underneath the bar and place it on your traps. You know, those big meaty pieces of muscle on top of your back. Now you're under it, just stand up with it and take 2 steps back and maybe a 3rd shuffle step to get your feet in position. Take a big belly breath and push your stomach out into the belt. Don't make the mistake of taking a big breath with your chest. When you do this your stomach muscles retract and you won't be able to brace against the belt as intended. Just think about inhaling a big breath and pushing it all down into your stomach. Make a fat belly basically. It braces your core and provides tons of support to your midsection. Wearing a weight lifting belt helps out a ton with this movement. It's pretty much another layer of armor protecting you from possible injury.

Now that you've got the bar on your back and you know how to brace your core, perform the squat. When you finish a rep and get back to the top, release your breath and inhale for another rep. Now do another rep. Same thing when you get to the top, exhale your breath and reload for another. I think of my big belly breath as a "Full Tank" providing me with fuel to execute my lift. If I have already exhaled on the way down for a squat, I've wasted my fuel for power and I've greatly compromised my core musculature because now my back is much more vulnerable to injury. Just remember to refill your tank at the top of every rep. This goes for all other strength exercises too.

Your squat should be deep enough that your thighs are parallel to the floor. I prefer deeper than that to be honest but that's just me. I'm more flexible than most and can squat far past parallel and remain flat footed. I recommend squatting as deep as you comfortably can while keeping your heels on the floor. If you're struggling keeping your feet/heels on the floor, squat shoes will help with this tremendously because of its elevated heel.

Another cue to think about is keeping the barbell over mid foot during the entire lift. On the way down and on the way up. The entire time. This will keep your balance in check and insure the most efficient lift possible. Think about it, If you're squatting heavy weights and you get pushed towards your toes and all your weight is on your toes, you are off balance and expending energy just trying not to fall over. This is valuable energy wasted that should've instead been used for driving the barbell upwards in a straight line. If you keep the bar in balance over the middle of your foot, you'll know your balance is right and you'll perform the lift as efficiently as possible.

Once you're done with your set of squats, just walk forwards to the rack and let the bar hit the rack before you start lowering the bar to the rack. I've seen too many times where people are re-racking their bar and they try to aim the bar into the j-hooks and miss completely. Without a spotter present this is potentially disastrous. So take my advice and make sure you hit the rack with the bar and then squat/lower the weight down onto the j-hooks.

The Bench Press

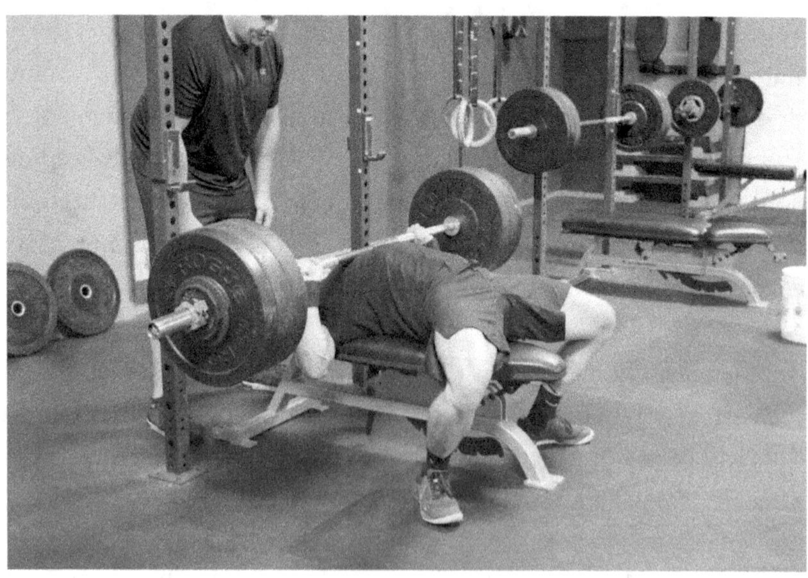

This has got to be most lifters favorite exercise. I can't lie, it's certainly one of mine too. This exercise arguably puts on more muscle mass in the upper body than any other lift out there. It mainly builds the chest and triceps. But among that, the upper back and legs are also involved if we want to be serious about putting up heavy weights.

Start by lying on the bench with your eyeballs directly underneath the bar. I've seen too many times people naturally lay down too far up on the bench. This might seem more natural at first, but when the person unracks the weight and goes to execute the lift, the bar hits the j-hooks/rack on the way up and it will fuck your day up badly if you don't have a spotter. So trust me, keep your eyes directly under the bar when unracking it.

Now go ahead and unrack the bar. Bring the bar out over your chest with your arms fully extended. This is called the "Lockout" position. Take a big breath just like in the squat. Remember, an empty tank is weak. A full tank is strong. Always fill your tank before you perform the movement. Once you've got your breath, bring the bar down to your chest under control. For most people, the perfect spot to touch the bar is right at the nipple line. It might sound weird but that's how it is. To avoid developing the bad habit of bouncing the bar off your chest, a good cue to remember is to think of your chest as a piece of glass. If you hit it too hard it's going to shatter. Just lightly tap your chest with the bar, then press the weight back up.

Another thing to remember is to always keep your eyes focused on the ceiling, not the bar. When you're in the lockout position before you lower the weight, stare at the ceiling with the barbell in your secondary vision. Notice where the bar is in relation to the ceiling? That's where you want to press the bar every time you do a rep. This will ensure you always hit the correct spot on your chest and you'll also lockout the weight in the correct spot. Think of throwing a baseball or football. You keep your eyes focused on where you want the ball to go. You don't look at the ball when you're in the process of throwing it. If you did, it would look very silly and your accuracy would be terrible. So just remember, look at where you want the bar to go. Don't follow the moving bar with your eyes. Also, your grip width should be that when the bar is touching your chest, your forearms are lined up vertically under the bar. This helps us become more efficient and train our muscles to their full extent.

The last two things I'll talk about for the bench press are re-racking the bar and safety clips. When you're finished with your set and ready to rack the bar, make 100% sure your arms are locked out. Then simply bring the bar towards the rack with your arms locked out. Once you've hit the rack right above the j-hooks you can lower the bar into the j-hooks. I've had quite a few personal training clients get in a hurry to rack the weights when they've finished a heavy set. They attempt to rack it before they've completed the rep and I scold them for it. Lightly of course. The critical point is this…. If you don't have a spotter to help you out, you could end up with a barbell in your mouth and your teeth aren't going to like it too much.

Safety clips for bench pressing. If you are benching with a partner or have a spotter by all means use them. I mean they help keep the weights on the bar so they are pretty useful. The problem arises when a person is bench pressing alone in their garage. Lets pretend you're benching alone in your home gym and you've got safety clips holding your weights on. And you can't lock out the bar and it's stuck on your chest. What the fuck do you do? Well to be honest you might be in big trouble. Quite a few deaths have happened in this scenario. So let's avoid that and keep the clips off the bar.

Keeping the clips off the bar allows you to dump the weights onto the floor and is a legitimate life saving technique. So say you're benching and you fail the rep and the bar comes back down on your chest. Don't panic. Just simply tilt the bar to one side and the weights will slide off that end. Then tilt to the other side and the weights will slide off. And now youre still alive.

The Deadlift

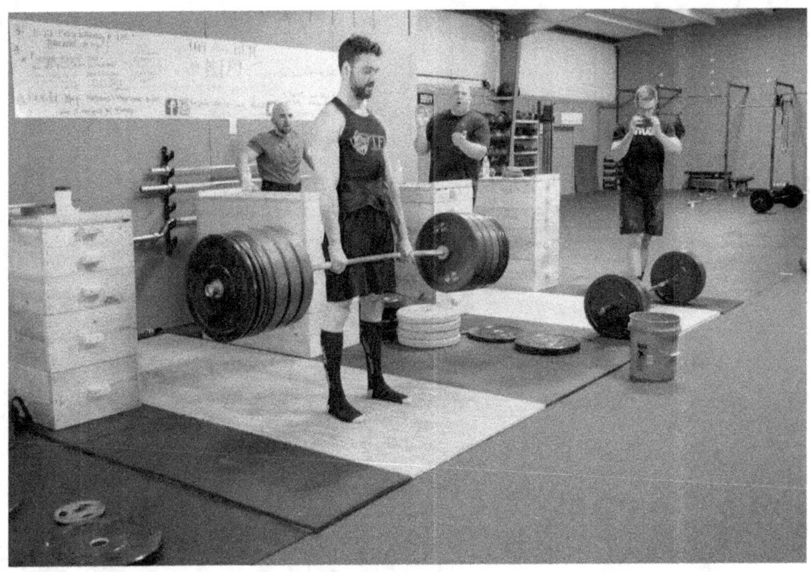

No other exercise trains more muscles in your body than the deadlift. It's at the top of the food chain for full body exercises. Your entire legs, butt, back, core, shoulders, arms, and hands get trained when performing deadlifts. The only thing it doesn't train is the chest but that's okay because everybody loves to bench press. Lots of people will skip training on squats and deadlifts for one main reason. They're hard! They require tremendous effort and focus. But the reward is a jacked physique, thick back, and serious full body strength.

To begin, place the barbell on the floor and load a pair of plates onto it. Most adult men should be comfortable starting with 135lbs which is a 45lb plate on each side. If you're unsure about your strength or have other reasons to start lighter (ie: an injury) then by all means start lighter. Remember though if you do start with something lighter, make sure the 10lb or 25lb plates you're using are full size in diameter just like the size of 45lb plates. This prevents you from bending over too far and putting your back in a compromised position.

I like to teach the 6 step process to set up for this lift:

Step 1: standing over the bar, look down and make sure the bar is lined up directly over the middle of your foot. This should put the barbell about 1" away from your shins.

Step 2: Hinge your hips backwards without bending your knees much at all. You should feel a stretch in your hamstrings if you're doing this right.

Step 3: Grip the bar with your hands, usually placed just outside your legs.

Step 4: Put your shins to the bar. Keep the bar still. Don't roll it to your shins. Bring your shins to the bar.

Step 5: Lift your chest upwards to flatten out and brace your back. This will take you from a rounded position to a stable, flat position.

Step 6: Pull! Execute the lift. Pay careful attention to dragging the bar right along your shins. It's uncomfortable but necessary. It'll save your back and allow you to lift heavier weights.

At the top of the lift, once again called the lock-out, you should be squeezing your butt cheeks. This helps ensure you get great leg drive. When lowering it, keep the bar close to you just as you did on the way up. More injuries happen deadlifting when lowering it vs when on the way up. So, don't baby the weight too much on the way down. Keep your core braced and lower it quickly.

And as always, gather a giant belly breath and have a full tank of air before you pull the weight off the floor. A weight-lifting belt is highly recommended when deadlift. Just use the same breath technique and push your belly into the belt. The last tip I'll give is make sure your knees don't cave inwards when pulling the weight up. Think "knees out" when lifting the weight. This helps get your glutes engaged and provides further leg drive.

The Overhead Press

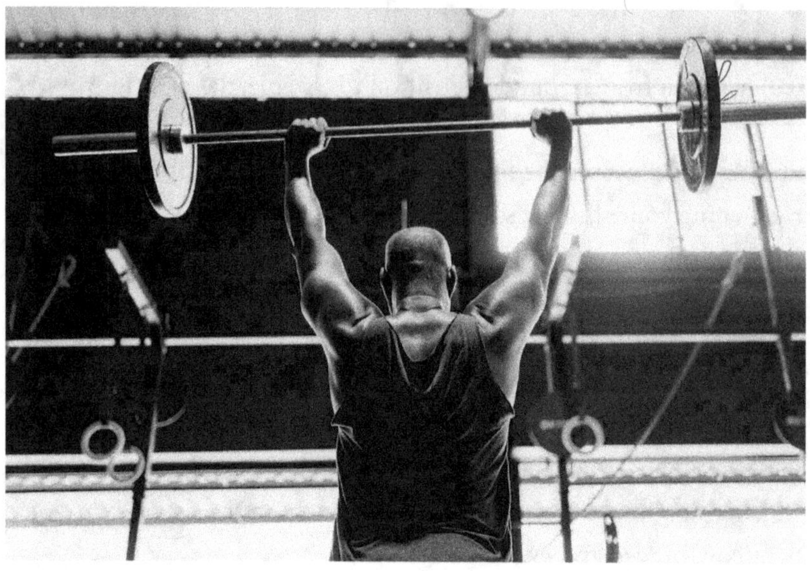

The overhead press or OHP as I like to abbreviate it, is an often overlooked exercise by many people. Lots of people seem to avoid it and just bench press all the time instead. Don't be one of them! The OHP promotes healthy shoulders, increases shoulder flexibility, gets your upper body seriously strong, and does one hell of a job of training your core.

Start with the barbell in the power rack. For most people, it'll be set as the same height as your squat setup. (about chest level) Walk under the bar, dip down a bit, and use your legs to pick the weight up. Don't stand away from the bar and grab it and bring it towards you. It's very inefficient.

Now that you've got the bar in your hands, take a step or two away from the rack. Your grip width will be narrower than your bench press width. When standing, your forearms should be vertical under the bar. Now get your breath, fill your tank up and press the weight overhead.

When pressing the weight, keep the bar as close to your face as possible without hitting it. If you move it out and away and then back up over your head you are losing lots of efficiency and won't lift nearly as much weight. Once the bar gets just over your head, drive your head under the bar and finish the lift by shrugging your shoulders. Think of it as you can't get the weight high enough and you're squeezing every bit of muscle in your traps to shrug the weight into lock out position. This should feel very secure and strong.

I've seen many people perform this lift and they never get their head under the bar. Instead they just press the weight up and away from them. And it quickly comes back down because there is never any true lockout.

One thing to note about the OHP is when to refill your tank of air. Most people naturally want to refill their breath at the bottom of the lift. But don't do this. When you've got the bar locked out overhead, that's when you refill your tank. Rinse and repeat this for every rep you do.

Keep your core braced and your glutes squeezed the entire time of this lift. It provides you a solid foundation to lift from. When you've finished your set, just walk back towards the rack and dip down by bending your knees and let the j-hooks catch the bar. That's it!

The Power Clean

The power clean along with the snatch can be very intimidating for people. In most public gyms you'll rarely see people doing them. It's not because they're extremely hard to do, but more so because they've never been taught how. And I'm here to teach you. Let's get started.

The power clean is a great full body lift that also trains your explosiveness. It's basically jumping with weight in your hands and catching it in "the rack" position. (Not to be confused with a squat/power rack). The rack position is where you find yourself at the bottom of the OHP. But instead, you rotate your elbows forward and try to get them as high as possible. This will shift the bar out of your hands and it'll roll onto your delts, with your fingers still underneath the bar.

So, start by picking up an empty bar. After you've deadlifted the bar to your hips and you're standing straight up, hinge over slightly and bend your knees a little bit. Don't lower it too much. Just 4 to 6 inches should be enough. When bending your knees, force them outwards and not straight forward. This keeps your balance over midfoot and makes for an optimal jump.

Now jump with the bar. Be sure to keep your arms straight when dipping and jumping and not prematurely bending your arms. Lots of people tend to do this and it will destroy your leg drive and jumping power. Now that you've jumped the bar into the air, catch it in the rack position on top of your delts. It's helpful and advisable to catch the bar in a slight dip position (called the receiving position) and not completely standing up straight. I call it "getting under the bar". Once you've caught the bar, you can stand up with it.

That's pretty much it for the power clean. Keep in mind, the stronger you get and as the bar gets heavier and heavier, you will not be able to jump the bar as high. So when you get to this point you'll have to start catching the bar lower and lower in the receiving position. Eventually you'll be catching it in the bottom of a front squat but that is out of scope for this book. I just want to get you started with this lift and not overwhelm you.

The Snatch

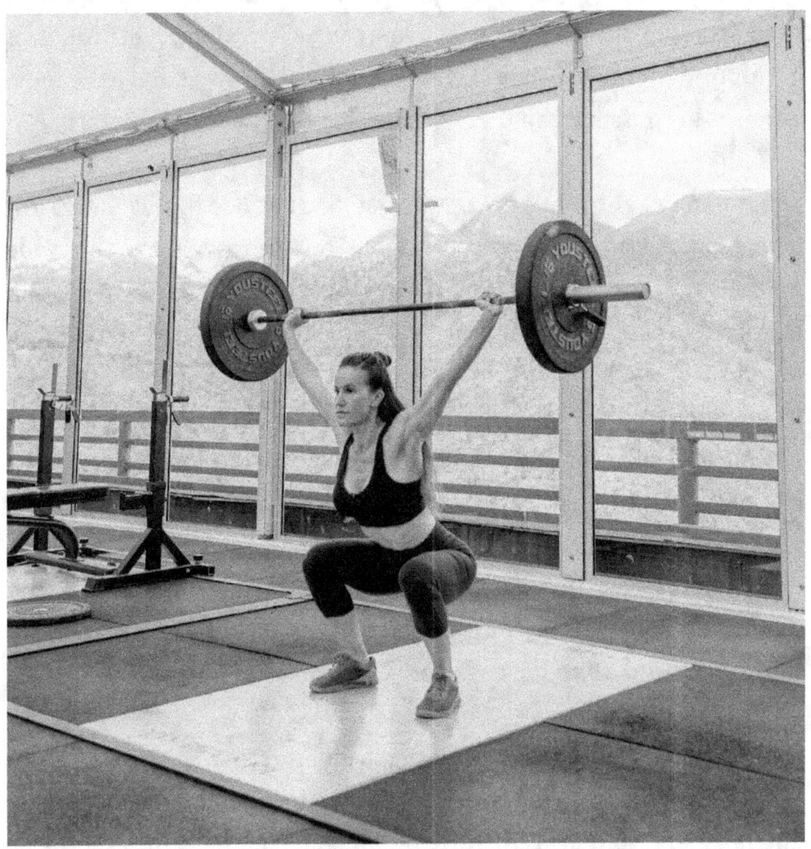

The snatch is the cousin of the power clean. I honestly found it easier to learn vs the power clean. The 2 key differences here are you hold the bar with a very wide grip and you jump with the weight and catch it overhead with locked out arms.

Your perfect grip width will place the bar at the crease of your hips when standing up straight. To find this, simply hold the bar with a snatch grip and lift one of your knees up. If the bar travels upward when you do this, you need to widen your grip. Keep playing with this setup until you get the bar right at your hip crease. This might seem like a pain in the ass step but we want to get as strong as possible right? Right. If we jump with the bar in line with our hip crease, we'll have the most efficient lift possible and therefore be able to lift heavier weights.

So now you've got your grip figured out. Start by deadlifting the weight with a snatch grip and stand up straight. Your arms should be very wide on the bar at this point. Now, dip down a little bit just like we did in the power clean. Bend your knees (driving them outwards, not directly forward) and bend over a tiny bit (hinge at the hips). Again, don't lower it too far down. Just enough where you feel you can get enough power to jump with the weight. 3" to 6" of downward bar travel should be enough. This is called "the jump" position.

Now, with the bar in contact with your hips (this is important. Don't jump with the bar away from your body. Keep it close or touching your hips), jump and catch the bar over your head. While doing this, make sure you keep your arms straight and locked out when dipping to the jump position and when performing the jump. People tend to be more patient on this lift vs the power clean in terms of maximizing leg power and not using your arms to move the weight. And I feel the exact same way. For some reason, the foreign nature of this extremely wide grip on the bar allows us to fully trust our legs and hips to move the weight. This is pretty awesome.

After you've jumped and are about to catch the bar overhead, try to dip or "pull" yourself underneath the bar a little bit. Then stand all the way up straight with your arms locked out. Also, think about shrugging your traps as hard as you can towards the ceiling. At this moment, you should feel like a badass. There is something empowering about doing a perfect snatch and holding the weight over your head.

Just as with the power clean, when the weight gets heavier and heavier, you won't be able to jump the bar as high. So, you'll gradually have to catch or "receive" the bar at lower heights. Eventually catching it all the way in the bottom of an overhead squat. Then just stand up with it and feel like Hercules.

If you have bumper plates on the bar (those rubber bouncy ones) you can drop the weight from overhead when you're done. If you're using iron plates, please don't drop it from this high. The plates and possibly the floor will break. So with iron plates, I like to catch the bar at my hip height (standing straight up with a snatch grip position) and dip down simultaneously to absorb the impact of the weight. Then lower it to the floor from there.

9

Other Important Exercises

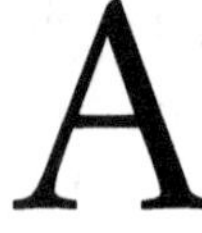

Aside from the big 6 barbell lifts, I'm going to list talk about my favorite accessory exercises.lifts. These are...

-Chin ups

-Pushups

-Row (barbell, kettlebell, or dumbell)

-Farmer carries (simply walking while holding heavy weights)

-Lunges (bodyweight or weighted)

-Sleds (pushing, pulling, etc.)

-Planks

-Turkish Get-Ups (a fantastic core and full body exercise)

-Ab Wheel

-Kettlebell swings, kettlebell snatches, kettlebell cleans, and kettlebell presses overhead

10

How To Plan a Workout

Okay, so now you know about the important lifts but you still need to know how to implement them into a training program. I like to advise most people to workout 3 to 4 days per week if increasing strength is your main goal. Far too many people insist on going 5 or 6 days per week because they're "Hardcore". This might be okay for weight loss or bodybuilding, but for developing maximal strength, it's not going to give you enough time to recover. Remember, adequate resting is crucial for gaining muscle and strength.

Let's begin with an every other day approach. This will get you into the gym 3.5x per week on average. And in my opinion, that's a perfect amount of training to rest ratio. And every workout we will be training our full body. There's no leg day, arm day, shoulder day, or build Frankenstein's arm pit day in this program. I like to train the body as one whole unit, using full body exercises every single workout.

The Program

Rest 3 minutes between each set for optimal recovery.

Monday- Day 1

-Squat 3 sets x 5 reps
   -Bench press 3 to 4 sets x 5 reps
   -Power clean 5 sets x 3 reps

Wednesday - Day 2

-Deadlift 2 to 3 sets x 4 reps
   -Overhead press 3 sets x 5 reps
   -Snatch 8 sets x 2 reps

Friday - Day 3

(add 5 lbs to what you did on monday)

-Squat 3 sets x 5 reps
   -Bench press 3 to 4 sets x 5 reps
   -Power clean 5 sets x 3 reps

Sunday - Day 4

(add 5 lbs to what you did on wednesday)

-Snatch 8 sets x 2 reps
   -Overhead press 3 sets x 5 reps
   -Deadlift 2 to 3 sets x 4 reps

You can rinse and repeat this program for quite some time and continue getting stronger without adding much of anything else. Squat day is workout A and deadlift day is workout B. Just keep rotating between those.

After you've been on this program for a while or you're already an experienced lifter, you can begin to add some of the accessory lifts I mentioned in the previous chapter. Just make sure you do them after the main lifts. And you don't need to add much. Here is a sample workout I would recommend...

Workout A

-Deadlift
   -Bench press
   -Snatch
   -Chinups (3 sets x AMAP) (As many as possible)

Workout B

-Squat
   -Overhead press
   -Power clean
   -Farmer carries (do 3 to 5 sets of max distance carries)

You can swap exercises and choose to bench press on your squat day and overhead press on your deadlift day. And you can power clean or snatch on either workout A or B. It doesn't matter. Just don't change anything else!

That's it! Easy huh? Continue working the program for 4 to 6 weeks and if you feel like you need another exercise then you can add one more. Just never add more than one thing at a time. Test out what you're adding one by one. This is smart training.

This workout would look like this...

Workout A

-Squat
  -Bench press
  -Snatch
  -Chinups
  -Lunges (bodyweight or weighted) 3 sets x 7 reps per leg

Workout B

-Deadlift
  -Overhead press
  -Power clean
  -Farmer carries
  -AB wheel (3 sets x 5 to 10 reps) (these are hard!)

Warming up

Warming up is pretty straight forward. You need to get your body warm. Wearing a sweatshirt and sweatpants if it's cold where you live is a great idea. Cold muscles are not as forgiving as warm muscles. This makes them much more prone to injury so let's avoid that.

You can get warm by walking an incline treadmill, exercise bike, rowing machine, etc. for 5 to 10 minutes. Another way is to sit in the sauna for a few minutes before your workout. This is really nice when it's cold outside.

Now that we've gotten our bodies warm, let's start our workout by performing each lift with the empty bar for 5 to 8 reps (except the deadlift, keep plates on this to maintain proper height from the floor). Continue to add small weight increments and slowly lower the amount of reps for each successive warm up set. Here's an example…

A person who has a max 5 rep squat of 225 lbs

-Squat the empty bar for 5 reps (all barbells are 45 lbs)
  -Squat with 95 lbs for 5 reps
  -Squat with 145 lbs for 3 or 4 reps
  -Squat with 185 lbs for 2 or 3 reps

And this person's working weight will be 215 lbs. So he/she will be lifting 215 lbs x 5 reps x 3 sets.

The idea here is to slowly acclimate the body to the weight. If you go cold turkey to the gym and squat 200lbs right away, it's going to feel like quite a shock because you went from squatting 0 lbs to 200 lbs. But if we gradually squat with increasing weights, and keep the reps low to avoid fatigue, we will be in the best shape to handle whatever is coming next!

11

Eating For Strength

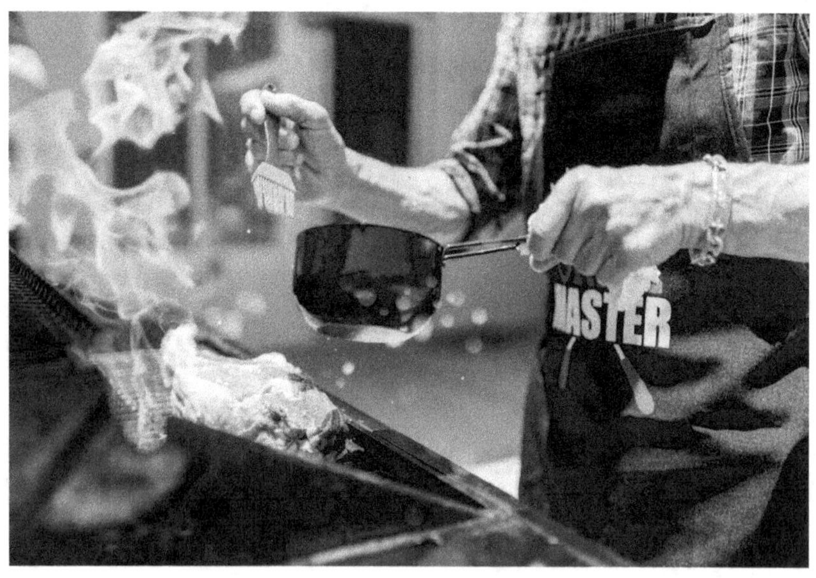

Y ou can't grow stronger if you don't eat. No matter how many times you go to the gym each week. Food is fuel. Think of it as such from now on. Your body is a race car and you need the best fuel possible to win the race. I'm going to keep this chapter simple and straight to the point. Eat lots of meat and vegetables. For your carbohydrate food source, I recommend rice and potatoes. They are easy to cook and will help fuel your workouts and help your body recover from previous workouts.

All lifters need protein. And lot's of it. It's a good idea to aim for 1 gram of protein per 1 pound of body weight. So, a 175 lb person should target 175 grams of protein per day. And if strength or muscle growth has stalled, increase it to around 200 grams. If you get in your protein requirements, the fats and carbohydrates will usually remain pretty low.

Here are some good food choices with high protein content…

-Eggs
  -Beef
  -Chicken
  -Pork
  -Fish
  -Protein powder
  -Whole milk
  -Peanut butter
  -Cheese
  -Nuts
  -Beans

Water is also a key factor in keeping our bodies in peak condition. I'd recommend 8 to 16 cups daily (½ gallon - 1 gallon). So keep eating and drinking water like a madman if you are serious about getting strong! Remember the 4 steps to strength: Lift weights, drink water, eat plenty of good food, and sleep your ass off! Aim to get 8 to 10 hours of sleep per night. Our bodies recover greatly when we get deep, restful sleep.

12

Conclusion

Well you've made it this far and I sincerely want to thank you for reading my book. I hope you've enjoyed it and find the information useful. I've been a strength coach for 10 years, however this is the first book I've written on the subject. I'm sure if you follow these principles you will make it very far in your weight lifting journey. I'll be writing more in depth books about strength and health in the future. Thanks again and I hope your life is better and stronger because of this book!

Please send any training questions to mattdalefitness@gmail.com
  -**Matt Dale**